Adrenal Fatigue Diet

A Beginner's Step-by-Step Guide to
Reversing Adrenal Fatigue Symptoms
Through Diet: With Recipes and a Meal Plan

mf

copyright © 2019 Brandon Gilta

All rights reserved No part of this book may be reproduced, or stored in a retrieval system, or transmitted in any form or by any means, electronic, mechanical, photocopying, recording, or otherwise, without express written permission of the publisher.

Disclaimer

By reading this disclaimer, you are accepting the terms of the disclaimer in full. If you disagree with this disclaimer, please do not read the guide.

All of the content within this guide is provided for informational and educational purposes only, and should not be accepted as independent medical or other professional advice. The author is not a doctor, physician, nurse, mental health provider, or registered nutritionist/dietician. Therefore, using and reading this guide does not establish any form of a physician-patient relationship.

Always consult with a physician or another qualified health provider with any issues or questions you might have regarding any sort of medical condition. Do not ever disregard any qualified professional medical advice or delay seeking that advice because of anything you have read in this guide. The information in this guide is not intended to be any sort of medical advice and should not be used in lieu of any medical advice by a licensed and qualified medical professional.

The information in this guide has been compiled from a variety of known sources. However, the author cannot attest to or guarantee the accuracy of each source and thus should not be held liable for any errors or omissions.

You acknowledge that the publisher of this guide will not be held liable for any loss or damage of any kind incurred as a result of this guide or the reliance on any information provided within this guide. You acknowledge and agree that you assume all risk and responsibility for any action you undertake in response to the information in this guide.

Using this guide does not guarantee any particular result (e.g., weight loss or a cure). By reading this guide, you acknowledge that there are no guarantees to any specific outcome or results you can expect.

All product names, diet plans, or names used in this guide are for identification purposes only and are the property of their respective owners. The use of these names does not imply endorsement. All other trademarks cited herein are the property of their respective owners.

Where applicable, this guide is not intended to be a substitute for the original work of this diet plan and is, at most, a supplement to the original work for this diet plan and never a direct substitute. This guide is a personal expression of the facts of that diet plan.

Where applicable, persons shown in the cover images are stock photography models and the publisher has obtained the rights to use the images through license agreements with third-party stock image companies.

Table of Contents

Disclaimer — 3
Table of Contents — 5
Introduction — 6
Chapter 1: Understanding the Adrenal Fatigue — 8
    Causes of Adrenal Fatigue — 10
    Lifestyle Changes and Medical Treatments for Managing Adrenal Fatigue — 11
Chapter 2: What is the Adrenal Fatigue Diet? — 13
    Basic Principles of Adrenal Fatigue Diet — 14
    Benefits of Adrenal Fatigue Diet — 16
    Disadvantages of Adrenal Fatigue Diet — 18
    Foods to Eat — 20
    Foods to Avoid — 21
Chapter 3 – Week 1: Your Preparation Stage — 23
    Step 1: Planning and Assessing — 23
    Step 2: Write down your medical statistics. — 24
    Step 3: Write down how you feel every day. — 26
Chapter 4 – Week 2: Making Small Changes — 27
    Step 1: Committing to a Time — 27
    Step 2: Replacing One or Two Meals a Day — 28
    Step 3: Prepare Everything You Need in Advance — 29
    Step 4: Create a List of Possible Adrenal-Friendly Quick Food Sources — 30
    Step 5: Make Conscious Diet Decisions — 32
    Step 6: Reassessing Your Status — 33
    Step 7: Compare and Eliminate — 34
Chapter 5 - Week 3: Flipping More Meals — 36
    Step 1: Replace another meal — 36
    Step 2: Repeat Recording and Assessing — 37

Chapter 7 – Repeat and Experiment with Other Adrenal Fatigue Diet Recipes to Try Out — **38**

    Salmon with Avocados and Brussels Sprouts — 38

    Adrenal Fatigue Coach Broth — 40

    Breakfast Scramble — 42

    Black Burgers with Avocado Buns — 43

    Baked Salmon — 45

    10-Minute Breakfast Hash With Plantains and Chimichurri — 46

    Adrenal Fatigue Diet Smoothie — 48

    Black Bean Hemp Burgers — 48

    Tempeh Kale Taco Salad — 50

    Sweet Potato Breakfast Bowl — 51

    Mediterranean Chicken Salad — 52

Chapter 8: 7-Day Sample Meal Plan — **54**

    Day 1 — 54

    Day 2 — 54

    Day 3 — 55

    Day 4 — 56

    Day 5 — 56

    Day 6 — 57

    Day 7 — 57

Conclusion — **58**

FAQs — **60**

Resources and Helpful Links — **62**

Introduction

If you're constantly feeling exhausted despite getting sufficient sleep, or find yourself frequently depending on caffeine or energy drinks to get through the day, it's possible you may be experiencing what's known as adrenal fatigue. But don't worry - addressing this could be as straightforward as tweaking your diet.

The Adrenal Fatigue Diet isn't merely a temporary dietary trend. It's a recognized nutritional strategy with a specific aim in mind - to tackle the root cause of your tiredness, which is your adrenal glands. These tiny yet vital organs are located above your kidneys and produce several important hormones that regulate energy levels, the immune system, and blood pressure, among other things. When their function is disrupted due to stress or poor nutrition, symptoms such as persistent fatigue, body aches, unexplained weight loss, and low blood pressure can occur.

The objective here is to change your morning routine. The goal is to wake up feeling refreshed and energized, without needing to depend on caffeine or sugar for an energy lift. The Adrenal Fatigue Diet aims to nourish and revitalize your adrenal glands, promoting their proper function and improving overall health.

By including certain nutrient-rich foods in your diet and avoiding others that can induce stress, you're supplying your body with the necessary nutrients it requires to recover and flourish. And there's no need to sacrifice flavor. The Adrenal Fatigue Diet includes a wide range of tasty and satisfying options to keep your meals interesting and your body well-nourished.

In this guide, we will talk about the following;

- Understanding The Adrenal Fatigue
- Causes, Symptoms, Lifestyle Changes, and Medical Treatments to Manage Adrenal Fatigue
- Understanding Adrenal Fatigue Diet
- Principles, Benefits, and Disadvantages of Adrenal Fatigue Diet
- Steps to Get Started with the Diet
- Foods to Eat and to Avoid
- Sample Recipes and Sample Meal Plan

Are you ready to seize back your energy and live life to the fullest once again? Stick with us as we delve deeper into the Adrenal Fatigue Diet - its components, the supporting science, and how you can easily blend it into your lifestyle. We'll also share success stories from individuals just like you who have transformed their lives through this powerful dietary approach.

If you're tired of the constant fatigue, take the first step today by reading on. Embrace the journey towards health and vitality - you absolutely deserve it!

Chapter 1: Understanding the Adrenal Fatigue

What are adrenal glands?

Before we talk about the Adrenal Fatigue Diet, it's important to first talk about the gland at the center of it all: the adrenal glands. These glands are located on the top of each kidney and are responsible for the production of hormones. Hormones are an important substance that controls practically everything about a person from their health, their rate of growth, emotions, mood, and sex.

Problems with the adrenal gland may be the cause of various health problems including Addison's Disease, Cushing's Syndrome, Adrenal Cancer, Congenital Adrenal Hyperplasia, and more.

People with adrenal gland problems often have the following symptoms: nausea, sweating, excessive fatigue, dizziness, increased salt cravings, low blood sugar, low blood pressure, dark skin patches, weight gain/loss, muscle and joint pain, and irregular periods.

What is Adrenal Fatigue?

Adrenal Fatigue is a complex condition that occurs when the adrenal glands, which are responsible for producing and regulating various hormones in the body, fail to function properly due to chronic stress. This can result in inadequate production or insufficient quantities of essential hormones, leading to a wide range of symptoms.

The underlying cause of Adrenal Fatigue lies in the fact that prolonged and intense stress can push the adrenal glands into overdrive. As a result, the glands become fatigued and struggle to maintain their normal functioning. This fatigue affects not only the production of hormones but also the overall ability of the adrenal glands to carry out their vital roles in the body's stress response system.

By understanding the intricate relationship between chronic stress, adrenal function, and the development of Adrenal Fatigue, we can better appreciate the importance of managing stress levels and supporting adrenal health. Taking proactive steps to reduce stress, practicing self-care, and seeking appropriate medical guidance can help restore balance to the adrenal glands and promote overall well-being.

Accordingly, signs that you have Adrenal Fatigue include but are not limited to the following:

- Constant tiredness
- Having problems going to sleep or problems waking up in the morning
- Unexplained weight loss
- Cravings for sweet or salty food items

- Digestive problems such as diarrhea, constipation, bloating, gas, cramping, and others
- Reliance on coffee and other stimulants to help push you through the day
- Acne breakouts
- Low libido
- Quickly getting hungry after eating
- Increases instances of being sick
- Brain fog and memory problems
- Irritability

If you experience all of this after going through a rough time or even if you just feel as though you've been working for far too long without a break, then chances are you are suffering from Adrenal Fatigue.

Causes of Adrenal Fatigue

Understanding the causes of adrenal fatigue is vital in managing this condition. Here are some factors that can contribute to adrenal fatigue:

- **Chronic Stress**: Prolonged periods of stress can overtax the adrenal glands, which are responsible for managing the body's stress response. Over time, this can lead to adrenal fatigue.
- **Poor Sleep**: Lack of quality sleep can contribute to adrenal fatigue. The adrenal glands need rest to

function optimally, and without it, they may become overworked.
- **Poor Diet**: Consuming a diet high in sugar, caffeine, and processed foods can put additional strain on the adrenal glands, potentially leading to adrenal fatigue.
- **Overuse of Stimulants**: Regular use of stimulants, such as caffeine and energy drinks, can cause the adrenal glands to produce excessive amounts of hormones, leading to eventual burnout.
- **Lack of Exercise**: Regular physical activity is essential for maintaining adrenal health. Without it, the adrenal glands may become less efficient at managing stress.
- **Exposure to Environmental Toxins**: Prolonged exposure to environmental toxins can put additional stress on the adrenal glands, potentially contributing to adrenal fatigue.

While the concept of adrenal fatigue is still a topic of debate among medical professionals, these potential causes underscore the importance of managing stress, maintaining a healthy lifestyle, and avoiding environmental toxins to support overall well-being and adrenal health.

Lifestyle Changes and Medical Treatments for Managing Adrenal Fatigue

Managing Adrenal Fatigue involves implementing both lifestyle changes and medical treatments. These approaches work together to support the adrenal glands and reduce the impact of stress on the body.

Lifestyle Changes

Making positive lifestyle changes is crucial for managing Adrenal Fatigue. Here are some suggestions for improving overall well-being and supporting adrenal health:

- **Prioritize Sleep**: Aim for 7-9 hours of sleep per night, and establish a consistent sleep schedule.
- **Follow a Balanced Diet**: Consume a diet rich in whole foods, including fruits, vegetables, lean proteins, healthy fats, and complex carbohydrates. Avoid processed foods and excessive amounts of sugar and caffeine.
- **Incorporate Stress-Reducing Activities**: Engage in stress-reducing activities such as meditation, yoga, deep breathing exercises, and spending time in nature.
- **Stay Hydrated**: Drink plenty of water throughout the day to support overall hydration and adrenal function.
- **Limit Stimulant Use**: Decrease or eliminate the use of stimulants such as caffeine and energy drinks to avoid overworking the adrenal glands.

Medical Treatments

In addition to lifestyle changes, there are also medical treatments available for managing Adrenal Fatigue. These treatments aim to support adrenal function and restore balance in the body. Some options include:

- **Hormone Replacement Therapy**: In cases of severe hormonal imbalances, hormone replacement therapy may be recommended to alleviate symptoms.
- **Adaptogenic Herbs**: Certain herbs, such as ashwagandha, rhodiola, and licorice root, are known for their ability to support adrenal function and reduce the impact of stress on the body.
- **Nutritional Supplements**: Nutritional supplements may be recommended to correct any nutrient deficiencies and support overall adrenal health.

These lifestyle changes and medical treatments can work together to help manage Adrenal Fatigue. However, it's crucial to consult with a healthcare professional before making any significant lifestyle changes or starting a new supplement regimen.

Chapter 2: What is the Adrenal Fatigue Diet?

The adrenal Fatigue Diet is a specific diet plan designed to support adrenal health and reduce the impact of stress on the body. It focuses on reducing inflammation, balancing hormones, and supporting overall well-being.

Basic Principles of Adrenal Fatigue Diet

Later on in this guide, we're going to give a week-by-week guideline on how to follow the Adrenal Fatigue Diet. Before doing that, however, it's important to understand the key principles concerning the Adrenal Fatigue Diet. All your dietary decisions should comply with all these principles. While we're going to first give you a weekly plan to help with your diet, you should be able to create your own as you notice the positive changes of AFD in your life.

Knowing your food sensitivities and intolerances

Some food items may be doing more harm than good to your body – even if they're generally accepted as healthy. For example, milk is often seen as a good source of calcium – but people with lactose intolerance find milk to be a bad addition to their diet. Hence, some food items are best left alone if they leave a bad taste in your mouth or your digestive system.

Eating food you're allergic to or are sensitive to factors in Adrenal Fatigue because your body has to work harder to digest and absorb the nutrients from this food. Hence – you suffer from digestive problems like inflammation, diarrhea, constipation, bloating, gas, and others. If you notice having these problems after eating certain food items, there's a chance that even if you're not allergic, you are slightly intolerant of them.

Knowing the best time to eat

The diet encourages eating every three hours. This helps keep your blood sugar within acceptable levels all through the day. Eating in between long periods causes the blood sugar to dip and causes more stress for the adrenals.

Keeping hydrated

Drinking 8 glasses of water a day is a fairly common principle – but you'll have to go the extra mile for AFD. Ideally, your water should be purified and filtered for any type of chemicals like chlorine. The pH should also be more base than acidic and of course, there should be no microorganisms inside it. Fortunately, purified water can be easily purchased nowadays and you can even install your water purifying system if you want.

Note that drinking too much water is just as bad because it dilutes electrolyte levels in the blood, which worsens the stress on your adrenal glands. Other sources of hydration should be weighed carefully. For example, you'd want to avoid fruit juices because of the high sugar content – even if the fruit juice is squeezed fresh. To fight off Adrenal Fatigue, you'd want to minimize the consumption of ALL sugar sources – including natural sugar. Fortunately, vegetable juices are fine and will provide you with the necessary nutrients without the excess sugar.

Cutting back on sugar and caffeine

Stimulants like sugar, coffee, and tea might seem good in the short term, but they lead to more stress on the adrenal glands as you kick start the energy before allowing it to dive down as sugar is consumed.

The goal is to keep that energy source strong and steady throughout the day so that the adrenal glands run smoothly without any unnecessary pressure. You will notice that by constantly seeking out stimulants, it also becomes remarkably easy for you to reach out for other sugar-raising snacks which adds further stress to the glands.

Add more protein and fat **to** *your diet*

Include more fish, nuts, and flaxseed in your diet to increase your intake of omega-3 and omega-6 fatty acids. Steer clear of saturated trans-fat which only adds to the overall stress of the glands. Good sources of protein include fish, fowl, dairy, eggs, and even plant sources.

Note though that these protein sources should come from unprocessed meat. Hence, sausages, hotdogs, bacon, and other prepackaged food items should be avoided. Vegetable protein sources include legumes, nuts, seeds, organic yogurt, and others.

Benefits of Adrenal Fatigue Diet

The Adrenal Fatigue Diet is designed to support your adrenal glands by providing them with the nutrients they need to function optimally. Here are some benefits of following this diet:

- **Boosts Energy Levels:** The diet is rich in complex carbohydrates, proteins, and healthy fats that provide a steady supply of energy throughout the day. This helps to combat the fatigue commonly associated with adrenal insufficiency.
- **Reduces Stress:** Certain foods in the diet, such as dark chocolate and green tea, contain chemicals that help to reduce stress hormones in the body. This can aid in the recovery of your adrenal glands.
- **Improves Sleep Quality:** The diet encourages the consumption of foods rich in magnesium and B

vitamins, which can help to improve sleep quality. Good sleep is essential for adrenal health.
- **Supports Immune System:** The Adrenal Fatigue Diet includes plenty of fruits and vegetables, which are high in antioxidants and other immune-boosting nutrients. This can help to protect your body from illness and infection.
- **Balances Hormones:** The diet is designed to stabilize blood sugar levels, which can help to balance hormone levels in the body. This is important for maintaining overall health and well-being.
- **Promotes Healthy Weight:** By focusing on whole, nutrient-dense foods and eliminating processed sugary foods, the Adrenal Fatigue Diet can help to promote a healthy weight.
- **Improves Mental Health:** Many of the foods included in the diet, such as fatty fish and nuts, are rich in omega-3 fatty acids. These have been shown to support brain health and improve symptoms of depression and anxiety.
- **Encourages Hydration:** The diet recommends drinking plenty of water and herbal teas, which helps to keep the body hydrated. Hydration is key for optimal adrenal gland function.

By following the Adrenal Fatigue Diet, you can provide your body with the necessary nutrients to support your adrenal glands and overall health. It's important to note that while this diet may be beneficial for those suffering from Adrenal Fatigue, it should not replace medical advice or treatment. Consult with a healthcare professional before making any significant changes to your diet.

Disadvantages of Adrenal Fatigue Diet

While the Adrenal Fatigue Diet offers a host of benefits, it's also important to acknowledge potential disadvantages:

- **Limited Food Choices**: This diet restricts certain foods such as sugar, soy, dairy, alcohol, gluten, and caffeine. This could limit meal options and potentially lead to nutrient deficiencies if not managed properly.
- **Overemphasis on Protein**: The diet suggests consuming between 20 and 30 percent lean proteins. While protein is crucial for health, too much protein could potentially cause issues like kidney damage, especially in individuals with pre-existing kidney conditions.
- **Difficulty in Adherence**: The diet requires strict adherence to specific food choices and eating times, which can be challenging for some people, particularly those with busy lifestyles or limited access to certain foods.
- **Initial Detox Symptoms**: As the body adjusts to the new eating pattern and reduced intake of processed

foods, some people might experience initial detox symptoms like headaches, fatigue, and irritability.
- **Risk of Misdiagnosis**: Adrenal fatigue isn't universally recognized as a medical condition. So if you're experiencing symptoms like chronic fatigue, it's essential to seek medical advice rather than self-diagnosing and trying to self-treat with a diet.
- **Lack of Scientific Evidence**: While anecdotal evidence supports the diet's benefits, there's a lack of scientific research affirming its efficacy in treating adrenal fatigue.

Despite these potential downsides, the benefits of the Adrenal Fatigue Diet could outweigh the disadvantages for many people. It focuses on nutrient-dense, whole foods and promotes balanced meals, which can support overall health. Remember, it's always best to consult with a healthcare professional before starting any new diet plan.

Foods to Eat

The Adrenal Fatigue Diet emphasizes nutrient-dense, whole foods that are easy to digest and have a healing effect on the body's stress response system. Here are some of the foods you should focus on:

- **Lean Proteins:** Foods like chicken, turkey, fish, eggs, and tofu provide essential amino acids for repair and regeneration in the body.
- **Healthy Fats:** Avocados, olives, coconut oil, nuts, and seeds are rich in healthy fats that provide sustained energy and help regulate blood sugar levels.
- **Leafy Greens and Vegetables:** Spinach, kale, broccoli, and other veggies are packed with vitamins and minerals that support adrenal health.
- **Whole Grains:** Foods like quinoa, brown rice, and oats provide slow-release carbohydrates that can help maintain steady energy levels throughout the day.
- **Fruits:** Berries, apples, and pears provide natural sweetness and are rich in antioxidants and fiber.
- **Seeds:** Flaxseeds, chia seeds, and sunflower seeds are high in nutrients that support adrenal health, including magnesium and vitamin B5.
- **Herbs and Spices:** Ginger, turmeric, and other anti-inflammatory herbs and spices can be beneficial.
- **Sea Salt:** Moderate use of sea salt is often recommended as adrenal fatigue can sometimes cause a drop in sodium and potassium levels.
- **Bone Broth:** Rich in nutrients and easy to digest, bone broth can be very soothing and healing.
- **Herbal Teas:** Herbal teas like licorice, ginseng, and green tea can help support adrenal health.

Remember, it's important to eat regularly to avoid blood sugar dips and spikes, which can put additional stress on your adrenals. It's also advised to pair proteins or fats with carbohydrates to help stabilize blood sugar levels. Always consult with a healthcare professional before starting any new diet plan.

Foods to Avoid

While following the Adrenal Fatigue Diet, there are certain foods you should aim to limit or avoid. These foods can cause inflammation, spike your blood sugar, or stimulate your adrenals in a way that could potentially exacerbate fatigue. Here's a list:

- **Caffeine:** While it might give you a quick energy boost, caffeine can overstimulate your adrenal glands and interfere with your sleep cycle.
- **Sugar and Sweeteners:** Foods high in sugar or artificial sweeteners can cause blood sugar spikes and crashes, which can put stress on your adrenal glands.
- **Alcohol:** Alcohol can disrupt your sleep and hydration levels, both of which are important for adrenal health.
- **Processed Foods:** Highly processed and fast foods often contain unhealthy fats, sugars, and additives that can lead to inflammation and stress in your adrenal glands.

- **Soy:** Some people with adrenal fatigue may find that soy worsens their symptoms, although the reasons aren't entirely clear.
- **Hydrogenated Oils:** Oils like vegetable and corn oil, which are high in trans fats, can promote inflammation and are best avoided.
- **High Potassium Foods:** With adrenal issues, the body sometimes struggles to balance potassium and sodium levels. So, it might be beneficial to limit very high-potassium foods like bananas and potatoes.
- **Dairy**: Some people may need to avoid dairy if they have an intolerance or allergy, as this can trigger an inflammatory response.
- **Gluten**: Similar to dairy, some people may need to avoid gluten if they have a sensitivity or intolerance.

Remember, everyone is unique, and what works for one person might not work for another. It's always best to listen to your body and consult with a healthcare professional to create a dietary plan that suits your individual needs.

Chapter 3 – Week 1: Your Preparation Stage

Once you've committed to health, you are ready to start the Adrenal Fatigue Diet. Week 1 can start on a Saturday, Sunday, or Monday – that's completely up to you. For best results, however, try to start this brand new road to health on a weekend as we'll go through the whole process on a step-by-step basis.

Step 1: Planning and Assessing

Your first day would consist of planning. That's all you will be doing – planning and assessing what you've done so far. Note that the Adrenal Fatigue Diet is not a "fad" diet that you can do in just 3 or 4 weeks and then stop. To keep your health consistently good, it's important to make many of the diet's principles as part of your lifestyle.

The first 7 days would be when you start a food diary. Grab a piece of notebook and start writing everything you eat during the day, what time you ate them, and what you feel afterward. The goals here are threefold: (1) your typical diet (2) your typical eating periods and (3) your sensitivity or allergies to these food items.

Why do you need to do this? Well, this should be done to provide you with a jump-off point. You won't be able to assess your improvement based on the Adrenal Fatigue Diet if you don't know how you started in the first place.

If you have a hard time writing down what you eat every day, just take a picture of the food before you eat it. This would give you not only the food you ate but also the time you ate it.

Step 2: Write down your medical statistics.

In this crucial second step, it's important to document your current medical statistics meticulously. This will serve as a solid foundation for understanding your health status before you embark on your journey with the Adrenal Fatigue Diet.

Begin by noting down key indicators of your overall health such as your blood sugar levels and blood pressure. These numbers can provide valuable insight into how your body is functioning internally. If you have access to past records, compare them to see if there are any significant changes or trends.

Next, focus on your energy levels. How would you rate them on a daily basis? Are you constantly feeling tired, or do you have enough energy to get through the day without feeling drained? Understanding your energy levels can help you gauge the stress on your adrenal glands and tailor your diet accordingly.

Pay attention to any physical discomfort you may be experiencing. Do you have any persistent aches or pains? If so, where are they located and what is their intensity? Documenting this information can help you identify if these symptoms improve as you progress with the diet.

Your body weight is another important statistic to record. It's not just about the number on the scale, but more about your body composition. Note any changes in weight distribution or muscle mass as you go along.

Lastly, keep track of your sleep patterns. How many hours do you sleep each night? Is your sleep restful or interrupted? Good quality sleep is essential for adrenal health, so any changes in your sleep pattern can be an indicator of improvements in adrenal function.

Remember, the goal here is to establish a clear baseline of your current health status. This way, you'll be able to measure your progress and see tangible proof of the positive changes that the Adrenal Fatigue Diet brings about in your health over time.

Step 3: Write down how you feel every day.

In this third step, it's essential to pay close attention to your feelings and emotions, as they can be significant indicators of Adrenal Fatigue. Symptoms such as lethargy, dizziness, and irritability are common, and keeping track of them daily can provide valuable insight into your progress.

Ideally, you should take a moment to pause and reflect on your feelings about an hour after each meal. This is the time when your body is actively digesting the food and the impact on your energy levels and mood can be most noticeable.

To make this process easier and more systematic, consider creating a rating scale from 1 to 10. Use this scale to quantify your feelings and symptoms. For example, if you're feeling particularly irritable, you might rate this feeling as a '7' on your scale. Likewise, if your energy levels are exceptionally low, maybe they would be a '2' or '3'.

This numerical system provides a clear, objective way to track changes over time. You can easily compare numbers from day to day and week to week, helping you identify patterns and trends. Are your energy levels generally higher on days when you eat certain foods? Does your irritability increase when you skip meals? These are the types of insights that can guide you in fine-tuning your Adrenal Fatigue Diet.

Remember, this step isn't just about tracking negative feelings or symptoms. Also, note when you're feeling good, energetic, or calm. These positive indicators are just as important and can serve as motivation to stick with your diet plan.

By consistently recording how you feel each day, you'll be creating a comprehensive, personalized map of your journey with the Adrenal Fatigue Diet. This will not only help you understand how different foods and eating patterns affect you but also empower you to make informed decisions about your diet and overall health.

Stick to this for 7 days. For the second week, the Adrenal Fatigue Diet starts.

Chapter 4 – Week 2: Making Small Changes

Step 1: Committing to a Time

As mentioned, eating every 3-4 hours is an important aspect of the Adrenal Fatigue Diet. That means that you'll be eating 4-5 small meals a day instead of 3 big meals. Here are the typical principles when deciding what kind of diet schedule you will set for yourself, depending on your situation:

- Always have your first meal before 10 AM, even if you're not hungry.
- Have your lunch early – perhaps around 11 AM. Hence, if you want your lunch around 11 AM, then your breakfast should be around 8 AM to maintain that 3-hour gap. You don't have to be so strict, however. You can try eating your breakfast around 6.30 AM, snacking around 9.30 AM and then having your lunch around 11.30 AM
- Cortisol levels start to dip around 3 PM to 4 PM. Hence, this is the best time to take your snack.
- Dinner should be around 5 PM to 6 PM.

You'll notice that this schedule doesn't jive with the typical workday of an individual. For example, your lunch hour may be 12 NOON to 1 PM and 6 PM might be too early for dinner. If you follow this dietary schedule without changing the quality of the food you eat – you're only going to cause additional fatigue to your adrenal glands. Hence, the next step is to make some changes to the food itself.

Step 2: Replacing One or Two Meals a Day

You can't be expected to change all your meals in one quick sweep. Going cold turkey not only makes the whole thing more difficult – but it also increases the chances of failure. Hence, it's better to make the changes small. For example, you can start with breakfast with this smoothie recipe:

Adrenal Healing Smoothie

- 12 ounces of full-fat coconut milk
- 1 tbsp. coconut oil or MCT oil
- 1 tbsp. maca powder
- 1 tsp. ashwagandha powder
- 1 tsp. Rhodiola powder
- 1 scoop collagen peptides
- 1 cup of frozen organic berries
- 1 cup spinach
- 1 drop stevia
- 5 brazil nuts

Just combine all these ingredients in the blender until they form a smooth and creamy mixture – perfect for a quick breakfast.

Step 3: Prepare Everything You Need in Advance

Perhaps the most difficult thing about following an Adrenal Fatigue Diet is the preparation. For example, the smoothie recipe given above requires an array of ingredients which can be confusing if you're new to creating smoothies. Hence, it makes sense to prepare food products in advance. For example, you can start chopping up vegetables and fruits and put them in the freezer.

This way, you can create a quick smoothie that's also the perfect temperature. With the above-given recipe, you also have the option of premixing all the dry ingredients together and simply adding the wet ingredients when in the blender. Since most powders are made to last for months, you can easily store them in the fridge without any problems.

You can also find simple Adrenal-friendly recipes if you prefer to eat something hot in the morning:

Adrenal-Friendly Porridge

- 1 cup boiling water
- 1 tbsp. chia seeds
- 1 tbsp. pumpkin seeds
- 1 tbsp. brown flaxseed
- 2 tbsp. unsweetened shredded coconut
- 1 tsp. cinnamon
- ¼ cup walnuts

- Salt to taste

Combine all the dry ingredients except salt and put them in a high-speed blender. Blend them all until finely grounded. Put the boiling water into the blender and start blending slowly. Gradually increase the speed until you get a smooth concoction. Place the porridge in a bowl and add salt to taste. You can garnish this with favorite toppings like coconut, sunflower seeds, and fruits. Try not to go overboard with the fruits however as this can contain sugar.

Step 4: Create a List of Possible Adrenal-Friendly Quick Food Sources

Unfortunately, preparation is not always possible – especially if you happen to have a busy schedule. Hence, it's also a good idea to have go-to restaurants or stores that will offer you adrenal-friendly food products. Unfortunately, the Adrenal Fatigue Diet isn't as popular at the same level as vegans or vegetarians. Hence, it's unlikely that you'll find restaurants that have a ready menu to meet your needs for reinvigorated adrenal glands.

So what do you do? Your first option is always to make or prepare your food yourself. If this is not possible, you have the option of keeping your dishes simple. Hence, you can choose to steam vegetables, pressure-cook meat, or even eat certain vegetables raw. Quick and handy snacks like nuts will also keep your blood sugar levels constant without necessitating extra work on your part.

Your third option – which should only be made if the other two are not available - is to buy meals from restaurants. The problem with this approach is that you will have less say in what goes into the food. There's no way you can monitor how much sugar or salt is placed in the product.

So this is what you do: you visit your favorite restaurants and start assessing the menu there. You remember what food items are as close as possible to an adrenal-friendly diet and make a list of them. This is your "emergency" list and when worse comes to worst, these are the places and food items you can tap to stay true to your Adrenal Fatigue Diet.

Step 5: Make Conscious Diet Decisions

In this fifth step, it's crucial to remember that every meal counts when you're on the Adrenal Fatigue Diet. It's not enough to eat one healthy meal and then let the rest of your day's food choices be dominated by less nutritious options. Every meal should be a conscious decision made with the health of your adrenal glands in mind.

This doesn't mean you have to banish all so-called "bad" foods from your diet immediately. Instead, consider gradually limiting their consumption. Adopting an all-or-nothing attitude can lead to feelings of deprivation and make it harder for you to stick to your diet in the long run. So, it's about finding a balance and making smarter substitutions where possible.

For instance, if you're accustomed to drinking three cups of coffee a day, try cutting down to just one. This simple reduction can significantly decrease the stress on your adrenal glands without making you feel like you're giving up something you enjoy.

Similarly, consider tweaking your favorite foods to make them healthier. If you love a caramel macchiato, could you reduce the sugar content? Small changes like this can add up over time without making you feel like you're sacrificing taste or enjoyment.

When it comes to carbohydrates, don't shy away from them entirely. Instead, opt for healthier alternatives. If bread is a staple in your diet, consider replacing it with nutrient-dense cereals or whole grains. These provide sustained energy release that can help support your adrenal function better than refined carbs.

Remember, the key here isn't about drastic dietary changes, but making conscious, mindful decisions about what you eat at each meal. This approach will not only benefit your adrenal health but also contribute to your overall well-being. By taking control of your diet in this way, you'll be taking a significant step toward overcoming Adrenal Fatigue.

Step 6: Reassessing Your Status

As you embark on the second week of your Adrenal Fatigue Diet plan, it's crucial to remember that this phase is essentially an extension of the first week, with only minor modifications to your routine. This means that you need to continue with the practices you established in the initial week: documenting what you eat, assessing how you feel post-meal, and recording your health status daily.

During this second week, the primary change will be in your meal plan. Aim to replace just one of your four or five daily meals with a more adrenal-friendly option. This could mean swapping out a high-sugar breakfast for a protein-rich alternative or replacing a caffeine-heavy afternoon snack with a nutritious smoothie.

If you're feeling confident and have adjusted well to the first week's changes, you may opt to modify two meals. However, be cautious about not overdoing it. Changing too much too soon can lead to feelings of overwhelm, making it more likely for you to abandon the diet altogether. The goal here isn't to make sweeping changes overnight but to gradually adapt your diet in a way that supports your adrenal health without causing undue stress.

Remember, this journey towards better adrenal health is a marathon, not a sprint. It's about making consistent, sustainable changes rather than drastic ones that are hard to maintain. So take it slow, listen to your body, and don't rush the process. The key is to build a healthier dietary routine that you can maintain in the long run, leading to lasting improvements in your adrenal function and overall well-being.

Step 7: Compare and Eliminate

As you conclude the second week of your Adrenal Fatigue Diet plan, it's time to take a comprehensive look at your dietary habits. Reflect on all the foods you've consumed over the past two weeks. Remember, in the first week, you took the initial step of replacing one meal – the easiest one for you – with an adrenal-friendly alternative. Maybe it was breakfast because you had ample time to prepare a nutritious start to your day.

Now, in this step, your task is to critically assess your diet from the second week and identify the least healthy food or drink you consumed. This could be anything from a pack of French fries to a couple of cans of Coke. Whatever it is, acknowledge this as your most significant dietary misstep for the week.

Going into your third week, commit to eliminating this unhealthy item from your diet. It's not about punishing yourself but rather making a conscious decision to improve your dietary habits for the betterment of your adrenal health.

But how do you eliminate this item? The solution lies in substitution. Replace this unhealthy choice with a healthier alternative. If you're used to reaching for a can of Coke, consider swapping it with a refreshing smoothie or a glass of freshly squeezed lemon juice. Both options are not only healthier but also provide essential nutrients that support your adrenal function.

Remember, the goal here isn't to make drastic changes overnight but to gradually shift towards healthier eating habits that support your adrenal health. By identifying and eliminating your least healthy choices one at a time, you'll be making significant strides toward improving your overall well-being and managing Adrenal Fatigue more effectively.

Chapter 5 - Week 3: Flipping More Meals

Step 1: Replace another meal

At the end of the second week, you identified your worst transgression, committed to eliminating it from your diet, and replaced it with a healthier option that's in line with your overall goal. During this time, you should also make a point of replacing another meal in your diet. Check out this Chicken Omelet recipe, which should be perfect:

Chicken Omelet (2-3 servings)

- 8 eggs
- 1 tbsp. olive oil
- 1 tsp. chili powder eggs
- ¼ cup of water
- ½ cup of water
- ½ cup diced tomatoes, seeded
- 1 cup cooked chicken, chopped into chunks
- Cooking fat
- Salt and pepper to taste

Start by putting ½ cup water with the olive oil, the tomatoes, and the chili powder in a high-speed blender. Process the combination until you get a smooth puree. Bring a saucepan into slow heat and pour the puree until you get a smooth and consistent simmer. Allow it to thicken for 7 minutes. Add some salt and pepper to taste. When you're happy with the taste, slowly add the chicken and mix. The chicken is already pre-cooked so you're just making sure it blends well with the puree. Lower the heat.

Crack the eggs open into a ¼ cup of water and whisk them all together. Season with salt and black pepper to taste. Grab a pan and put some cooking fat into it. Now start pouring a bit of the egg mixture slowly, gently moving it with a spatula for that perfect runny omelet look. When done, add the sauce and fold. You can make multiple omelets from the 8 eggs so feel free to partition the omelet and the sauce.

Step 2: Repeat Recording and Assessing

Moving forward, your journey is all about consistency and repetition. The practice of recording what you eat, how you feel afterward, and the time you consume your meals should become a part of your daily routine. This mindful approach towards eating can help you understand your body's reactions to different foods and identify any patterns that emerge.

Remember, it's not just about jotting down what's on your plate. It's equally important to note your physical and emotional responses after each meal. Do you feel energized or sluggish? Satisfied or still hungry? These details can provide valuable insights into how your current diet is affecting your overall well-being.

At the end of every week, set aside some time to review your food diary and evaluate your progress. Reflect on the changes you've made and assess how they're impacting your health. Are the healthier meals making a difference? Are you feeling better overall? This weekly reassessment will give you a clear picture of your journey so far and help you understand where you stand in your pursuit of better adrenal health.

By consistently documenting and assessing your dietary habits, you'll be able to make more informed decisions about your diet, tailor your meals to better suit your needs, and ultimately, take greater control of your adrenal health. Remember, the key to success lies in repetition and consistency. Keep going, and don't lose sight of your ultimate goal – improved well-being and a healthier you.

Chapter 7 – Repeat and Experiment with Other Adrenal Fatigue Diet Recipes to Try Out

Here are other Adrenal Fatigue Diet recipes you can try out!

Salmon with Avocados and Brussels Sprouts

Salmon preparation

- 2 pounds of salmon filet, cut into 4 pieces
- 1 tsp. ground cumin
- 1 tsp. paprika powder
- 1 tsp. onion powder
- 1 tsp. chili powder
- ½ tsp. garlic powder
- Himalayan sea salt
- Black pepper, freshly grounded

Avocado Sauce

- 2 chopped avocados
- 1 lime, squeezed for the juice
- 1 tbsp. extra-virgin olive oil
- 1 tbsp. fresh minced cilantro
- 1 diced small red onion
- 1 minced garlic clove
- Himalayan sea salt to taste

- Black pepper, freshly grounded

To cook this delicious dish, start by combining the cumin, onion, chili powder, garlic, and paprika seasoned with salt and pepper. Mix them well before dry rubbing it on the salmon. Place the salmon in the fridge for 30 minutes.

Preheat the grill. Grab a bowl and mash the avocado inside it until you get a smooth texture. Pour in all the remaining ingredients and mix thoroughly. Grab the salmon from the fridge and grill it for 5 minutes on each side or until cooked. Drizzle the avocado on your cooked salmon.

Brussels Sprout

- 3 lbs. of Brussels Sprout
- ½ cup raw honey
- ½ cup balsamic vinegar
- ½ cup melted coconut oil
- 1 cup dried cranberries
- Himalayan sea salt to taste
- Black pepper, freshly grounded

Preheat the oven to 375 degrees Fahrenheit. Now mix the Brussels Sprouts with the coconut oil and season them with salt and pepper. Place the vegetables on a baking sheet and roast them for about 30 minutes. In a separate pan, combine the vinegar and honey. Simmer them in slow heat until it boils and thickens. Drizzle them on top of the Brussels Sprout.

Adrenal Fatigue Coach Broth

Ingredients:

- 4 lbs. mixed beef bones
- 2 medium carrots, chopped
- 2 medium onions, chopped
- 3 celery stalks, chopped
- 1 tbsp. coconut oil
- 2 tbsp. apple cider vinegar
- 1 bay leaf
- Peppercorns to taste
- Salt, to taste
- Garlic, optional

Instructions:

1. Preheat your oven to 400 degrees Fahrenheit. Put the bones in a roasting pan and drizzle it with coconut oil or olive oil.
2. Roast for 30 minutes and then flip them over before roasting the other side for 30 minutes.
3. Take the bones out and put them in a large soup pot. Add the vinegar, vegetables, bay leaf, salt, garlic, and peppercorns.
4. Add 10 cups of water and turn on the heat to a high simmer. Once it's boiling, reduce the heat and allow it to simmer for 12 to 24 hours. Check every hour and

add more water to make sure that all the ingredients remain submerged in water.
5. Once you get that rich brown color, you can use a cheesecloth to remove all the remaining solid ingredients.
6. The broth should be allowed to cool until room temperature. After this, you can put it in the fridge and serve it as needed upon reheating. Make sure to remove the fat off the surface before you reheat.

Breakfast Scramble

Ingredients:

- 15 oz. can of chickpeas
- ½ tsp. salt
- ½ tsp. turmeric
- ½ tsp. pepper
- ½ white onion diced
- 2 cloves garlic, minced
- Virgin olive oil, to drizzle

Instructions:

1. Begin by preparing your ingredients. Dice half a white onion and mince two cloves of garlic.
2. Drain and rinse the chickpeas thoroughly under cold water.

3. Once drained, transfer the chickpeas to a bowl and mash them using a fork or a potato masher until you achieve a slightly chunky texture.
4. Heat a drizzle of virgin olive oil in a non-stick skillet over medium heat.
5. Add the diced onion to the skillet, stirring occasionally until it becomes translucent and begins to soften. This should take about 3-5 minutes.
6. Next, add the minced garlic to the skillet and continue to stir for another minute until the garlic is fragrant.
7. Sprinkle the salt, turmeric, and pepper into the skillet and stir well to evenly distribute the spices.
8. Add the mashed chickpeas to the skillet and mix everything together. Cook for about 5-7 minutes, stirring occasionally until the chickpeas are heated through and have absorbed the flavors of the spices.
9. Remove the skillet from the heat. Your breakfast scramble is ready to serve! Enjoy it as is, or pair it with your favorite breakfast sides like toast or fresh fruits.

Remember, cooking times may vary slightly based on your stove's heat and the type of skillet used. Always keep an eye on your dish to prevent overcooking or burning. Enjoy your nutritious and flavorful breakfast scramble!

Black Burgers with Avocado Buns

Ingredients:

- 4 avocados
- Tomatoes
- Salsa
- Salad greens
- 15.5 ounces of black beans
- 2 large cloves of garlic
- ½ red pepper
- ½ white onion
- ¼ tsp. of garlic granules
- 2/3 cup of gluten-free bread crumbs
- Salt and pepper

Instructions

1. Start by preparing the vegetables: Dice half a red pepper, half a white onion and two large cloves of garlic.
2. Drain and rinse the black beans thoroughly under cold water.
3. In a large bowl, mash the black beans using a fork or a potato masher until they are mostly broken down but still have some texture.
4. Add the diced vegetables, garlic granules, and gluten-free bread crumbs to the bowl with the mashed black beans. Season with salt and pepper to taste.
5. Mix all the ingredients together until well combined. If the mixture is too sticky, add more bread crumbs. If it's too dry, add a bit of water.

6. Shape the mixture into burger patties. The size of your patties will depend on the size of your avocados, as these will serve as your buns.
7. Heat a non-stick skillet over medium heat. Once heated, add the black bean patties and cook for about 5 minutes on each side, or until they are crispy on the outside and heated through.
8. While the patties are cooking, prepare the avocado buns. Cut the avocados in half and remove the pits. Slice a bit off the bottom of each avocado half to create a flat base.
9. To assemble the burgers, place one black bean patty on the bottom half of an avocado. Top with salad greens, sliced tomatoes, salsa, and finally, the top half of the avocado.
10. Repeat this process for the remaining black bean patties and avocados.

Baked Salmon

Ingredients:

- 2 salmon filets
- 6 cups of fresh spinach
- 2 tsp. coconut oil
- 1 tsp. coconut oil
- ¼ tsp. garlic powder
- ¼ tsp. turmeric

- 3 large cloves of garlic
- Lemon juice
- Salt and pepper to taste

Instructions:

1. Preheat your oven to 400°F (200°C).
2. Meanwhile, prepare the salmon filets. Rinse them under cold water and pat dry using a paper towel.
3. Season the salmon filets with salt, pepper, garlic powder, and turmeric.
4. Heat 2 tsp of coconut oil in a frying pan over medium heat. Once hot, add the salmon filets, skin side down. Cook for about 3-4 minutes until the skin is crispy.
5. Transfer the salmon filets to a baking tray and bake in the preheated oven for 10-12 minutes, or until the salmon is cooked to your liking.
6. While the salmon is baking, prepare the spinach. Heat 1 tsp of coconut oil in a pan over medium heat. Add the garlic cloves (finely chopped) and sauté until fragrant.
7. Add the fresh spinach to the pan and cook until wilted. Season with salt and pepper to taste.
8. Remove the salmon from the oven and squeeze some fresh lemon juice over the top. Serve the baked salmon on a bed of sautéed spinach.

10-Minute Breakfast Hash With Plantains and Chimichurri

Ingredients:

- 2 ripe plantains
- 2 cups of fresh parsley
- 2 cups of fresh cilantro
- 4 cloves of garlic
- 1/2 cup of olive oil
- 2 tablespoons of red wine vinegar
- 1/2 teaspoon of red pepper flakes
- Salt and pepper to taste
- 2 tablespoons of coconut oil

Instructions:

1. Start by peeling the plantains and cutting them into small cubes.
2. Heat the coconut oil in a skillet over medium heat. Add the plantain cubes and fry until they are golden brown and crispy, this should take about 5 minutes. Stir occasionally to prevent them from sticking to the pan.
3. While the plantains are cooking, prepare the chimichurri. Combine the parsley, cilantro, garlic, olive oil, red wine vinegar, and red pepper flakes in a blender or food processor. Blend until you have a smooth sauce. Season with salt and pepper to taste.

4. Once the plantains are done, remove them from the heat. Drizzle the chimichurri sauce over the fried plantains.
5. Serve your Breakfast Hash immediately while it's warm. Enjoy this delicious and quick breakfast!

Please note: The spiciness of the dish can be adjusted based on personal preference by increasing or decreasing the amount of red pepper flakes.

Adrenal Fatigue Diet Smoothie

Ingredients:

- 1 cup of fresh spinach
- 1 ripe banana
- 1/2 cup of blueberries (fresh or frozen)
- 1 cup of almond milk (unsweetened)
- 1 tablespoon of chia seeds

Instructions:

1. Begin by washing the fresh spinach thoroughly under cold water.
2. Peel the ripe banana and cut it into chunks.
3. If you're using fresh blueberries, wash them well. If you're using frozen blueberries, they can go straight into the blender.

4. In a blender, combine the spinach, banana chunks, blueberries, almond milk, and chia seeds.
5. Blend all the ingredients together until the mixture is smooth and creamy. This should take about 1-2 minutes depending on the power of your blender.
6. Once the smoothie is blended to your desired consistency, pour it into a glass.
7. Serve the Adrenal Fatigue Diet Smoothie immediately for the best taste and maximum health benefits.

Black Bean Hemp Burgers

Ingredients:

- 2 cans of black beans (drained and rinsed)
- 1/2 cup of hemp seeds
- 1 small onion (finely chopped)
- 2 cloves of garlic (minced)
- 1 teaspoon of cumin
- Salt and pepper to taste
- 1-2 tablespoons of olive oil

Instructions:

1. Start by preheating your oven to 375 degrees Fahrenheit (190 degrees Celsius).
2. In a large bowl, mash the black beans until they form a paste-like consistency.

3. Add the hemp seeds, chopped onion, minced garlic, cumin, and salt and pepper to the mashed black beans. Mix well until all the ingredients are combined.
4. Form the mixture into patties, about the size of a regular burger. This recipe should yield about 4-6 patties depending on how large you make them.
5. Place the patties onto a baking sheet lined with parchment paper. Drizzle or brush each patty with a bit of olive oil.
6. Bake the burgers in the preheated oven for about 15-20 minutes, or until the patties are firm and slightly crispy on the outside.
7. Once done, remove the burgers from the oven and let them cool for a few minutes before serving.
8. Serve your Black Bean Hemp Burgers on a bun with your favorite toppings, or enjoy them on a salad for a lighter meal.

These burgers are packed with protein from the black beans and hemp seeds, making them a great plant-based alternative to traditional meat burgers. Enjoy!

Tempeh Kale Taco Salad

Ingredients:

- 1 block of tempeh
- 2 cups of kale (washed and chopped)

- 1 can of black beans (drained and rinsed)
- 1 cup of cherry tomatoes (halved)
- 1 avocado (sliced)
- 1 teaspoon of cumin
- 1 teaspoon of chili powder
- Salt and pepper to taste
- 2 tablespoons of olive oil
- Your favorite salsa and vegan sour cream for topping

Instructions:

1. Start by heating the olive oil in a skillet over medium heat.
2. Crumble the tempeh into the skillet and add the cumin, chili powder, and a pinch of salt and pepper. Stir well to combine the spices with the tempeh.
3. Cook the tempeh for about 10 minutes, or until it's browned and crispy. Stir occasionally to prevent it from sticking to the skillet.
4. While the tempeh is cooking, prepare your salad base. In a large bowl, combine the chopped kale, black beans, cherry tomatoes, and sliced avocado.
5. Once the tempeh is done, add it to the salad bowl.
6. Top your salad with your favorite salsa and a dollop of vegan sour cream.
7. Toss everything together to combine the flavors and serve your Tempeh Kale Taco Salad immediately.

Sweet Potato Breakfast Bowl

Ingredients:

- 1 large sweet potato
- 1/2 cup of almond milk (unsweetened)
- 1 tablespoon of chia seeds
- 1/2 teaspoon of cinnamon
- A pinch of salt
- Toppings: sliced bananas, blueberries, a drizzle of almond butter, and a sprinkle of granola

Instructions:

1. Begin by washing the sweet potato thoroughly. Then, poke several holes in it with a fork.
2. Microwave the sweet potato for about 5-6 minutes, or until it's soft and cooked through. You can also bake it in the oven at 400 degrees Fahrenheit (200 degrees Celsius) for about 45 minutes.
3. Once the sweet potato is cooked, let it cool for a few minutes. Then, cut it in half and scoop out the flesh into a bowl.
4. Add the almond milk, chia seeds, cinnamon, and a pinch of salt to the bowl. Mash everything together until you get a smooth and creamy consistency. If the mixture is too thick, add a bit more almond milk.
5. Transfer the sweet potato mixture to a serving bowl.

6. Top your breakfast bowl with sliced bananas, blueberries, a drizzle of almond butter, and a sprinkle of granola.
7. Serve your Sweet Potato Breakfast Bowl immediately for a nutritious and energy-boosting start to your day!

Mediterranean Chicken Salad

Ingredients:

- 2 boneless, skinless chicken breasts
- 1 teaspoon of dried oregano
- Salt and pepper to taste
- 2 tablespoons of olive oil
- 4 cups of mixed salad greens (like romaine, spinach, or arugula)
- 1 cup of cherry tomatoes (halved)
- 1 cucumber (sliced)
- 1/2 red onion (thinly sliced)
- 1/2 cup of kalamata olives
- 1/2 cup of feta cheese (crumbled)
- Lemon vinaigrette dressing (1/4 cup of fresh lemon juice, 1/2 cup of olive oil, 1 clove of garlic minced, salt and pepper to taste)

Instructions:

1. Season the chicken breasts with the dried oregano, salt, and pepper on both sides.

2. Heat the olive oil in a skillet over medium heat. Add the chicken breasts and cook for about 6-7 minutes on each side, or until they're fully cooked and no longer pink in the middle. Once done, remove the chicken from the skillet and let it rest for a few minutes.
3. While the chicken is resting, prepare your salad. In a large bowl, combine the mixed salad greens, cherry tomatoes, cucumber slices, red onion slices, kalamata olives, and crumbled feta cheese.
4. Cut the rested chicken into thin slices and add them to the salad bowl.
5. To make the lemon vinaigrette, combine the fresh lemon juice, olive oil, minced garlic, salt, and pepper in a small bowl. Whisk until well combined.
6. Drizzle the lemon vinaigrette over the salad and toss everything together to combine the flavors.
7. Serve your Mediterranean Chicken Salad immediately, garnished with a bit more feta cheese if desired.

Chapter 8: 7-Day Sample Meal Plan

Day 1

Breakfast

- 10-Minute Breakfast Hash With Plantains and Chimichurri

Lunch

- Grilled chicken salad with olive oil dressing

Dinner

- Easy Chicken Casserole with Green Chiles

Snacks

- A handful of mixed nuts and seeds

Day 2

Breakfast

- Apple Pecan Quinoa Breakfast

Lunch

- Tempeh Kale Taco Salad

Dinner

- Vegetable stir fry with brown rice

Snacks

- Greek yogurt with honey

Day 3

Breakfast

- Avocado and Tomato on Whole Grain Toast

Lunch

- Chickpea Scramble Breakfast Bowl

Dinner

- Black Bean Hemp Burgers

Snacks

- A piece of Dark Chocolate and An Orange

Day 4

Breakfast

- Oatmeal with fresh fruit and walnuts

Lunch

- Tuna salad with olive oil dressing

Dinner

- Easy Chicken Casserole with Green Chiles

Snacks

- A banana and a handful of almonds

Day 5

Breakfast

- Greek yogurt with granola and blueberries

Lunch

- Chickpea salad with tomatoes and cucumbers

Dinner

- Crockpot Chicken and Cauliflower Rice Soup

Snacks

- An apple and a handful of walnuts

Day 6

Breakfast

- Apple Pecan Quinoa Breakfast

Lunch

- Chickpea Scramble Breakfast Bowl

Dinner

- Black Bean Hemp Burgers

Snacks

- Greek yogurt with a drizzle of honey

Day 7

Breakfast

- Oatmeal with sliced banana and almonds

Lunch

- Grilled chicken salad with olive oil dressing

Dinner

- Vegetable stir fry with brown rice

Snacks

- A piece of dark chocolate and an orange

Remember, the goal of the Adrenal Fatigue Diet is to eat nutrient-dense foods that help to support adrenal health. This includes lean proteins, complex carbs, and plenty of fruits and vegetables. You should also aim to stay hydrated throughout the day by drinking plenty of water and avoiding stimulants like caffeine and alcohol, as they can stress your adrenals.

Conclusion

Congratulations! You've made it to the end of this comprehensive guide on the Adrenal Fatigue Diet. It's a significant accomplishment, and your commitment to improving your health is truly commendable.

You've navigated through the science behind adrenal fatigue, understood its symptoms, and most importantly, you've learned about the dietary changes that can help manage and improve this condition. Remember, the journey to improved health is not a sprint but a marathon. It takes time, patience, and consistent effort.

By now, you should have a solid understanding of how food can serve as medicine for your body. Eating a balanced diet rich in lean proteins, complex carbohydrates, healthy fats, and plenty of fruits and vegetables can provide your body with the nutrients it needs to support your adrenal glands and overall health.

You've also learned about the importance of avoiding processed foods, caffeine, and sugars, which can exacerbate adrenal fatigue symptoms. While these foods may offer temporary satisfaction, they often lead to energy crashes that can leave you feeling worse in the long run.

One key takeaway from this guide is that managing adrenal fatigue goes beyond just diet. It's also about creating a lifestyle that supports your overall well-being. Regular exercise, adequate sleep, stress management, and staying hydrated are just as important as what you put on your plate.

Remember, everyone's body is unique and what works for one person might not work for another. It's important to listen to your body and adjust your diet and lifestyle accordingly. If you're unsure about anything, don't hesitate to reach out to a healthcare professional. They can provide personalized advice based on your specific needs and circumstances.

You should be proud of the steps you've taken so far. Learning about adrenal fatigue and how diet can impact it is the first step toward regaining control over your health. As you embark on this journey, remember to be patient with yourself. Change takes time and every small step you take is a move in the right direction.

In conclusion, the Adrenal Fatigue Diet isn't just a diet – it's a lifestyle change aimed at supporting your adrenal health and overall well-being. By making these changes, you're not only addressing adrenal fatigue but also paving the way for a healthier, more vibrant life.

Remember, it's not about perfection, but progress. Each meal is a new opportunity to nourish your body and support your health. So here's to celebrating the positive changes you've already made and to those yet to come. You're on the right track, and you've got this!

Thank you for taking the time to read this guide. We hope it has provided valuable insights and practical tips that will help you on your journey to better health. Keep going, stay positive, and remember - your health is worth fighting for!

FAQs

What is the Adrenal Fatigue Diet?

The Adrenal Fatigue Diet is a nutritional plan designed to support adrenal gland function and manage symptoms of adrenal fatigue. It focuses on nutrient-rich, whole foods and aims to reduce the intake of processed foods, caffeine, and sugar.

Can the Adrenal Fatigue Diet cure adrenal fatigue?

While there's no definitive 'cure' for adrenal fatigue, a balanced, nutrient-dense diet can help manage symptoms and support your body's overall health. The Adrenal Fatigue Diet aims to provide your body with the nutrients it needs to support adrenal function and reduce stress on these glands.

What foods should I avoid on the Adrenal Fatigue Diet?

Try to avoid processed foods, caffeine, alcohol, and high-sugar foods. These can cause spikes and crashes in blood sugar levels, which can stress your adrenal glands and exacerbate symptoms of adrenal fatigue.

Can I lose weight on the Adrenal Fatigue Diet?

While weight loss isn't the primary goal of the Adrenal Fatigue Diet, it could be a potential side effect. By focusing on nutrient-dense, whole foods and reducing your intake of processed and high-sugar foods, you may naturally consume fewer calories and lose weight. However, everyone's body responds differently, so individual results may vary.

Can I exercise while following the Adrenal Fatigue Diet?

Yes, regular, moderate exercise is beneficial for adrenal health. However, intense, prolonged exercise can stress the adrenal glands and may not be recommended if you're experiencing severe symptoms of adrenal fatigue. Always listen to your body and consult your healthcare provider if you're unsure.

Is the Adrenal Fatigue Diet suitable for vegetarians or vegans?

Yes, the principles of the Adrenal Fatigue Diet – eating nutrient-dense, whole foods and avoiding processed foods and high-sugar items – can be applied to any dietary preference. If you're vegetarian or vegan, focus on plant-based proteins, whole grains, fruits, vegetables, and healthy fats.

How long will it take to see results from the Adrenal Fatigue Diet?

Every person's body is different, so the time it takes to see improvements can vary. Generally, adopting healthier dietary habits and lifestyle changes can lead to noticeable improvements in energy levels and other symptoms within a few weeks. However, for some people, it may take longer. Be patient with your body and give it the time it needs to respond to these changes.

Resources and Helpful Links

Whitbourne, K. (2017, January 30). *Adrenal fatigue: Is it real?* WebMD. https://www.webmd.com/a-to-z-guides/adrenal-fatigue-is-it-real

Rd, R. a. M. (2021, October 1). *The adrenal fatigue (AF) diet*. Healthline. https://www.healthline.com/health/adrenal-fatigue-diet

Nd, M. J. (2023, November 3). *Adrenal fatigue diet — plans and foods to eat and avoid*. Women's Health Network. https://www.womenshealthnetwork.com/adrenal-fatigue-and-stress/the-adrenal-fatigue-diet/

Adrenal fatigue: What causes it? (2022, April 16). Mayo Clinic. https://www.mayoclinic.org/diseases-conditions/addisons-disease/expert-answers/adrenal-fatigue/faq-20057906

Foods for adrenal fatigue: What you should be eating & what you need to avoid. (2023, September 22).

https://www.healthieruny.com/resources/foods-for-adrenal-fatigue

Shomon, M. (2022, January 21). *What is adrenal fatigue?* Verywell Health. https://www.verywellhealth.com/adrenal-fatigue-exhaustion-3231648

Kirschner, L., MD PhD. (2023, March 21). *What is adrenal fatigue? Is it real?* Ohio State Health & Discovery. https://health.osu.edu/health/general-health/what-is-adrenal-fatigue

www.ingramcontent.com/pod-product-compliance
Lightning Source LLC
LaVergne TN
LVHW012036060526
838201LV00061B/4635